I Am Different, The Same As You

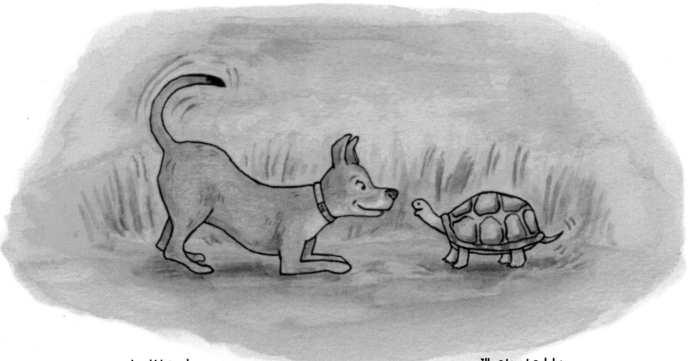

Written by
Deborah K. Okon

Illustrated by
Halsey Mollhagen

Illustration by
Halsey Mollhagen

Cover by
Tehsin Gul

ISBN: 9798852051653

Foreword

It's a real honor to be given the opportunity to write this Foreword for Debbie Okon's remarkable book for children, **I am Different, The Same as You**.

Debbie speaks to children much like St. Paul spoke to adults in 1 Corinthians, Chapter 12. The Apostle Paul taught us about the differences in people – each displaying different gifts, different styles, different backgrounds, and so forth.

In Romans 14, Paul tells us there are specific differences, even among genuine Christians. He explains that we must never take on a judgmental spirit toward others who seem peculiar or offbeat to us. It's true, we can hurt others who seem quirky to us by speaking to them (or about them) with loose or sarcastic words.

In this unique book, children will learn the importance of accepting and honoring people that seem different. Sometimes when a person looks a little different, they get teased or picked on by others. But Debbie explains to your children (in story form) why it's essential to be an encourager rather than a careless condemner.

This book is a winner if you're a parent, grandparent, or teacher. I have known Debbie Okon for nearly three decades. As a military person, she was featured in our "Stand Up for America Day" Celebration in Lansing, Michigan. She traveled as one of my team members to places like Minneapolis and Alexandria, Minnesota, Northern Michigan, and more. My wife and I have always found Debbie genuine, sincere, helpful, and kind. I fully endorse Debbie and her wonderful work for children **I Am Different, The Same as You!**

Dave Williams. D.Min, D.D.
Founder of the Center for Pacesetting Leadership

Dedication

I dedicate this book to my daughter, Stephanie, and my son-in-law, Curtis, for bringing Harlow into our lives. I have seen so much strength, dedication, and trust placed in your Lord Jesus Christ.

I am very proud of you both.

Proverbs 22:6
1 Thessalonians 5:17

Love,
Mom

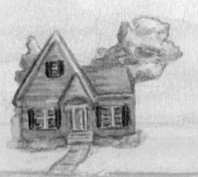

It was a warm, sunny day, perfect for walking to the river. Three friends, Harlow, Allen, and Olive, loved to watch the animals play in the river. Ollie, Harlow's dog, loved to see his friends at the river too.

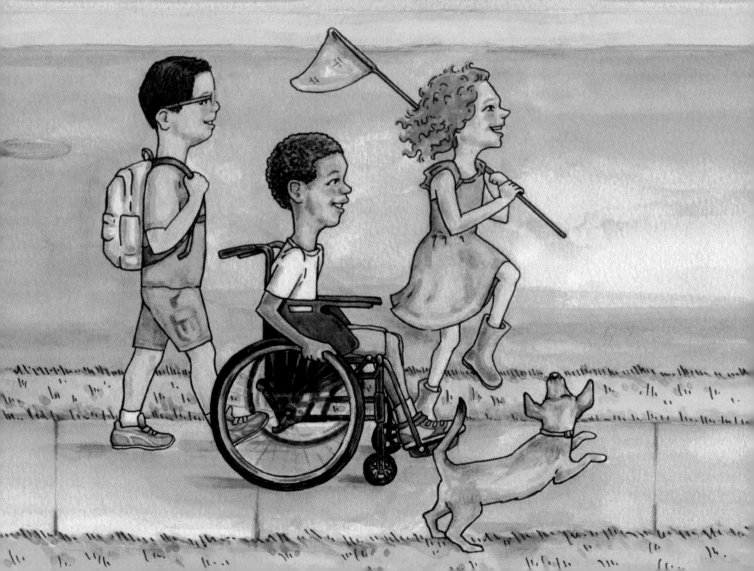

"Allen, do you want me to push you, or do you want to wheel yourself?" Harlow asked.

"My arms are tired," Allen answered as he hung his arms down, "I would like you to push me. Thanks."

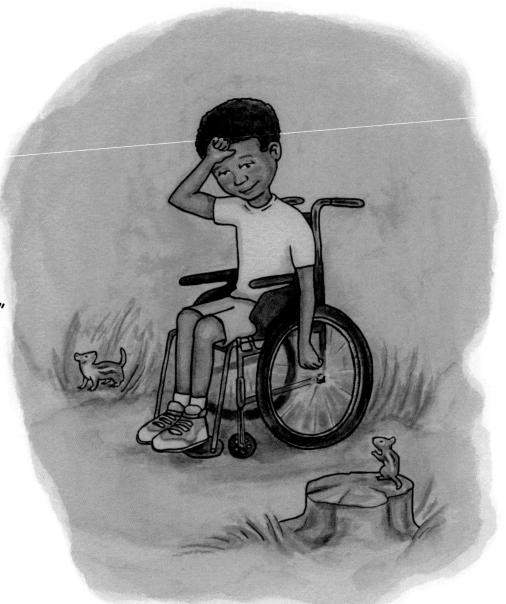

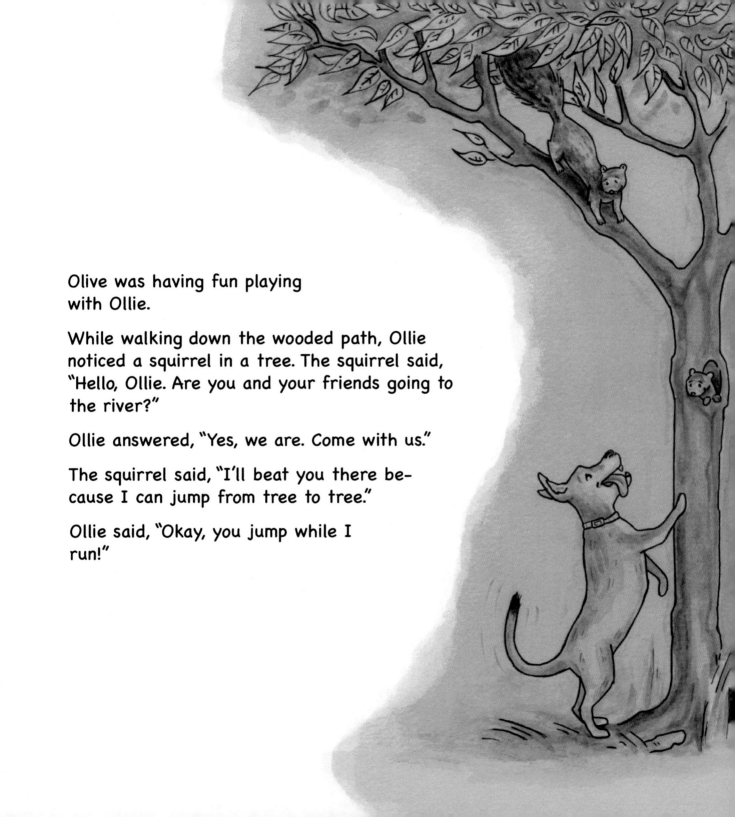

Olive was having fun playing
with Ollie.

While walking down the wooded path, Ollie
noticed a squirrel in a tree. The squirrel said,
"Hello, Ollie. Are you and your friends going to
the river?"

Ollie answered, "Yes, we are. Come with us."

The squirrel said, "I'll beat you there because I can jump from tree to tree."

Ollie said, "Okay, you jump while I
run!"

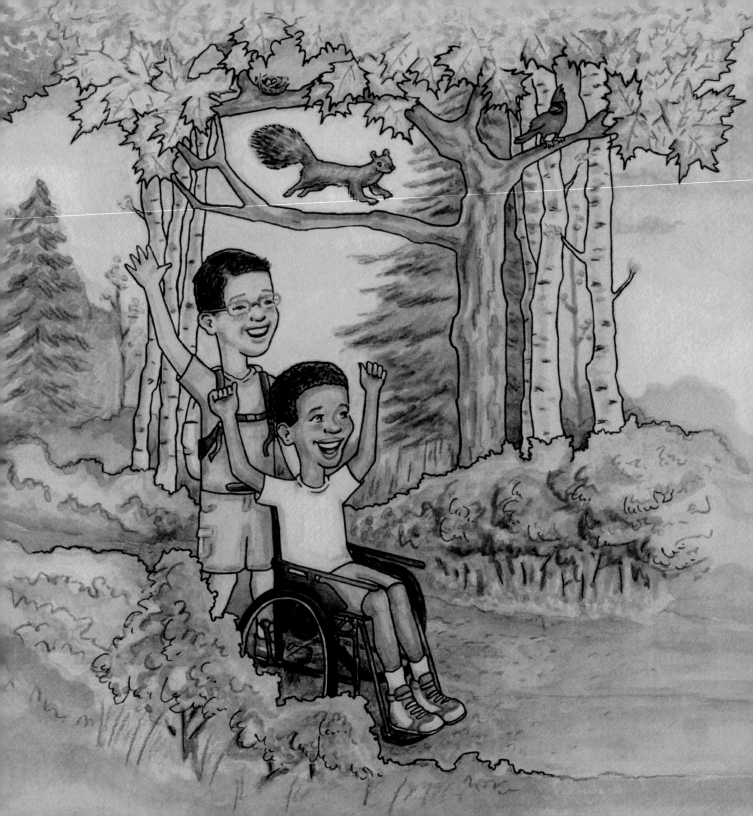

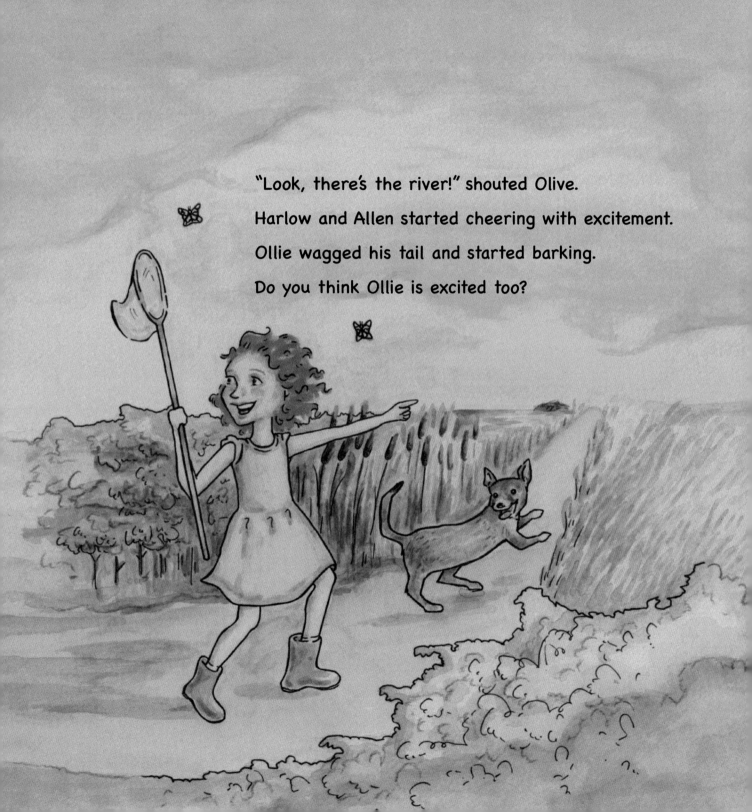

"Look, there's the river!" shouted Olive.

Harlow and Allen started cheering with excitement.

Ollie wagged his tail and started barking.

Do you think Ollie is excited too?

"WOW! The beavers are making a dam. It's fun watching them build it!" shouted Allen.

"Hey, did you know that beavers love sharing their home with the muskrat families?"

Olive answered, "Just like when we invite each other to our houses."

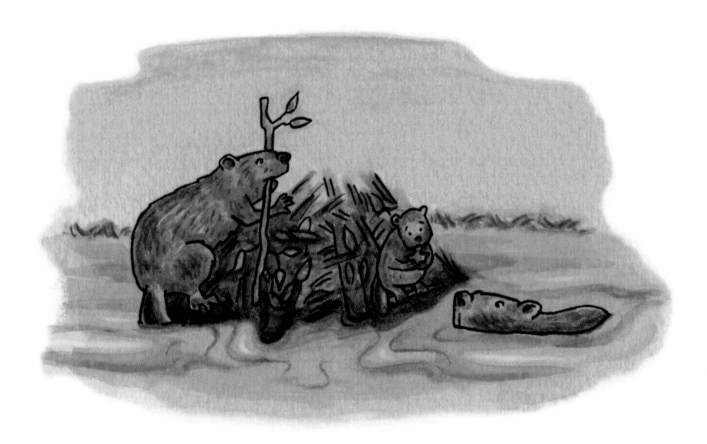

Then they saw a mama duck with her three ducklings following her.

Allen said, "Funny how they all stay in a straight line."

Harlow replied, "Ducks like to hang out with their duck friends. Like we are doing today."

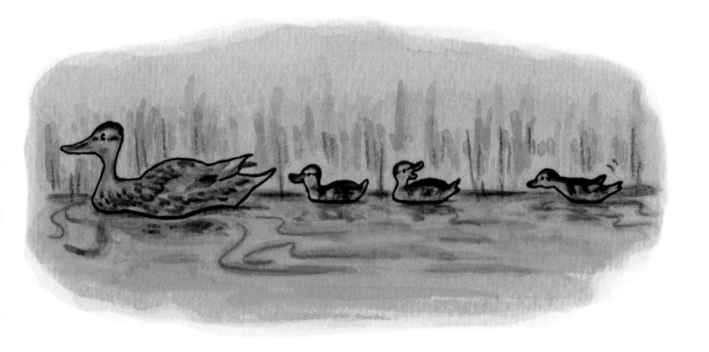

"WHOA, look at that otter," said Olive. "They always look like they have so much fun swimming."

Again Harlow shared, "Did you guys know that an otter can stay underwater for eight minutes? That's something ducks could never do!"

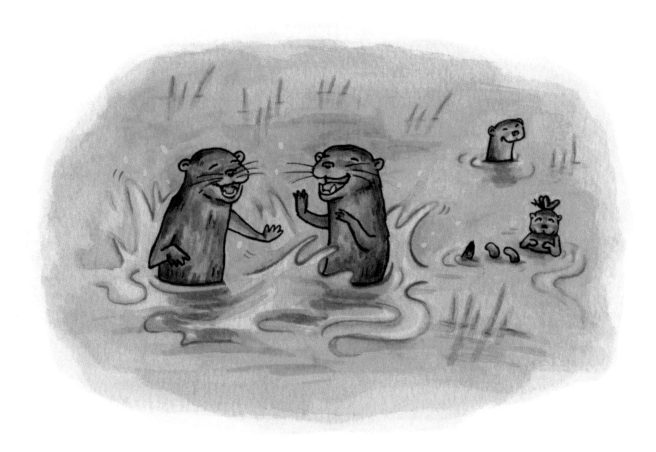

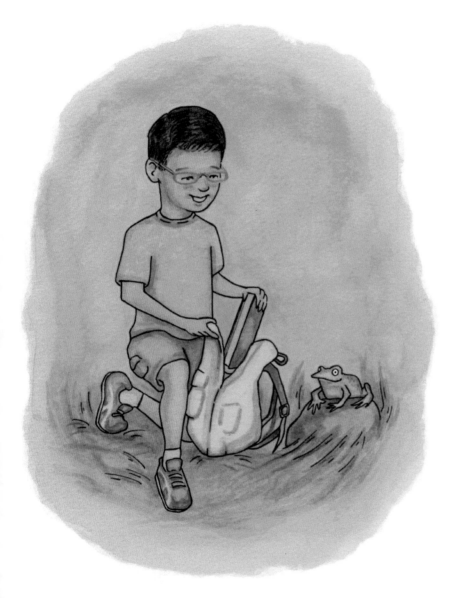

Allen asked, "Harlow, how do you know all these things about the beavers, ducks, and otters?"

"I read a lot. I like reading books because it helps me learn about things."

Allen said, "There's a turtle over there. I bet you don't know anything about turtles!"

Harlow explained, "Turtles do not have teeth."

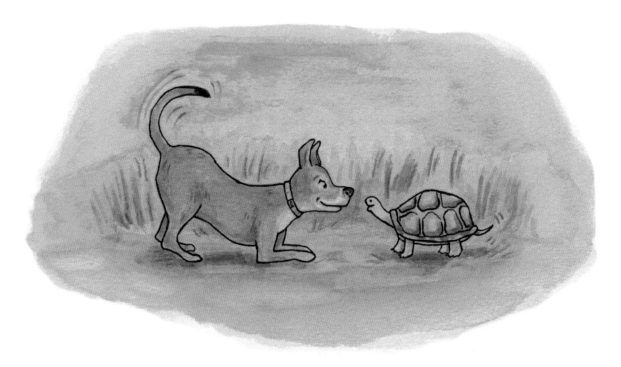

Olive was puzzled. "How do they eat food?"

"Turtles have sharp beaks. They use their beaks to cut their food," Harlow answered.

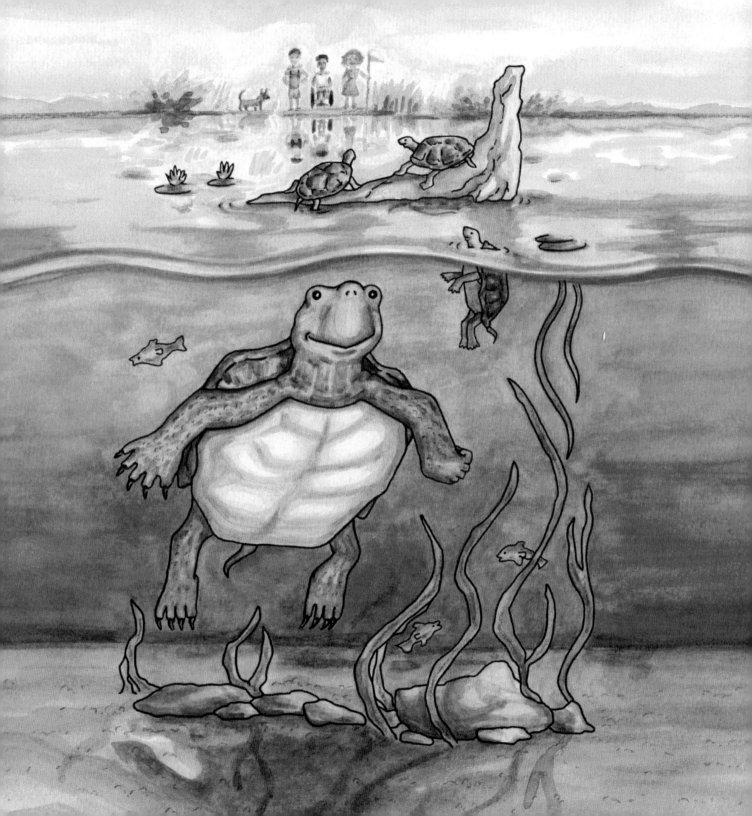

Olive said, "Look at all the river animals. Each one is different, and they all get along."

"Yeah, just like us. We are all DIFFERENT, and we get along. It is a lot of fun being different and playing together. I'm going to tell my friends that being different is okay." Allen said.

"Look, I'm in a wheelchair. That's different than using your legs to walk," Allen explained.

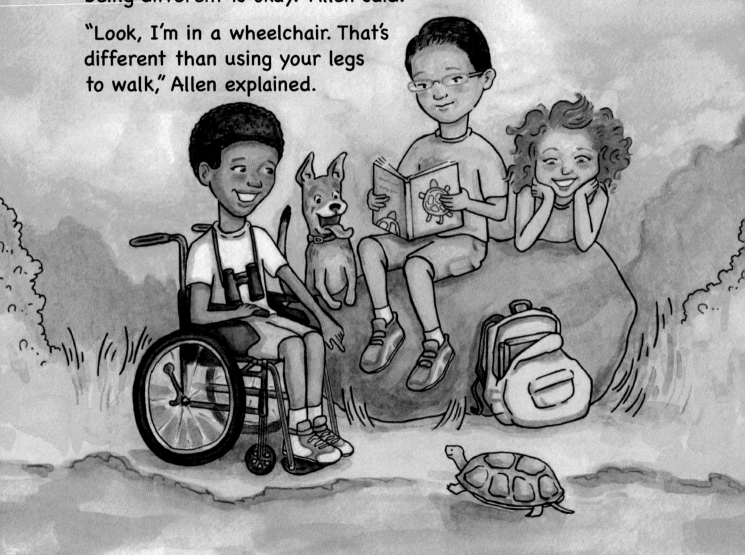

Olive said, "Look at me, I am a girl with red hair, and you are both boys. That is different."

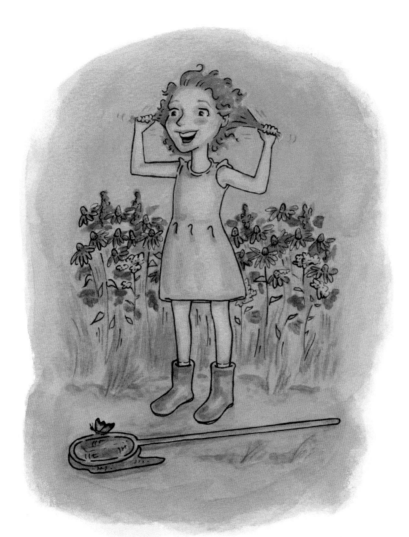

"Harlow, it's your turn. What is different about you?" asked Allen.

"When I was born, the doctor said I was a baby with Down syndrome. I am more like you than I am different. I love playing with my friends. I like reading. I love going on walks with my dog, Ollie. I love eating applesauce. With Down syndrome, I have to try harder to learn, which takes me longer sometimes, but I always get better each time I try."

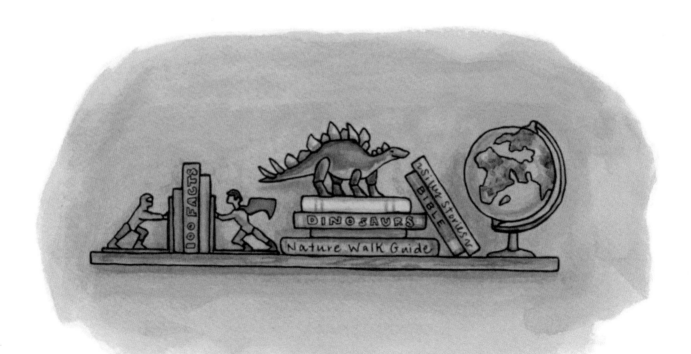

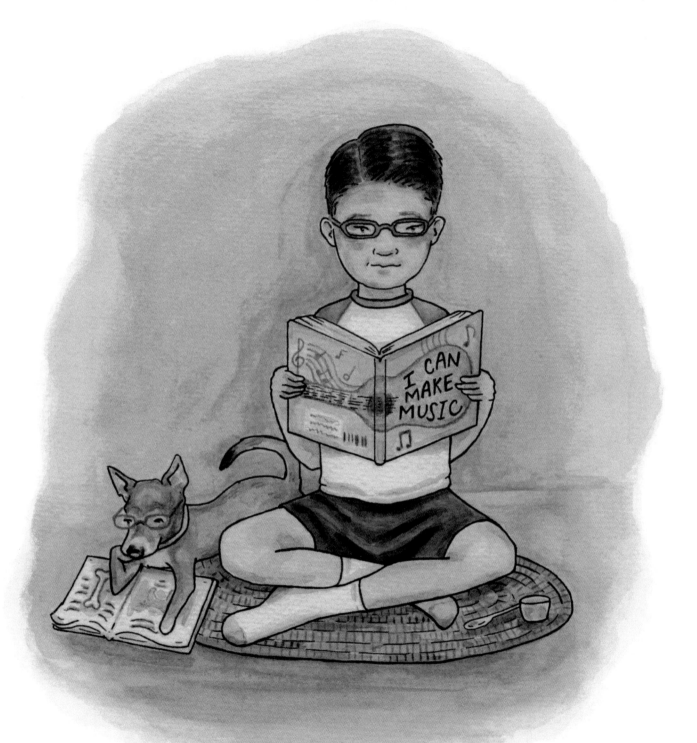

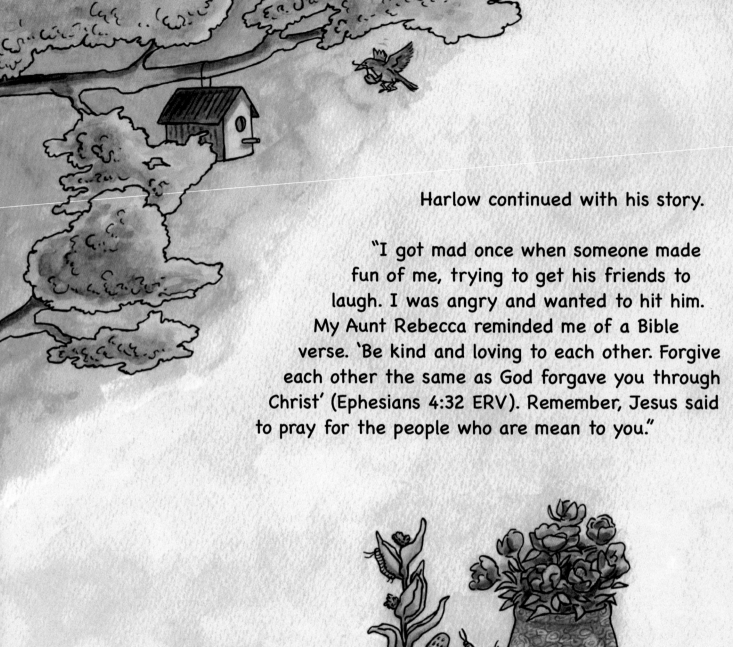

Harlow continued with his story.

"I got mad once when someone made fun of me, trying to get his friends to laugh. I was angry and wanted to hit him. My Aunt Rebecca reminded me of a Bible verse. 'Be kind and loving to each other. Forgive each other the same as God forgave you through Christ' (Ephesians 4:32 ERV). Remember, Jesus said to pray for the people who are mean to you."

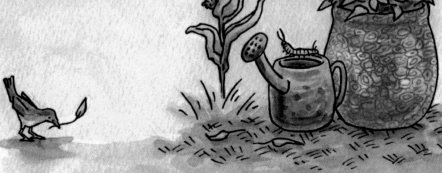

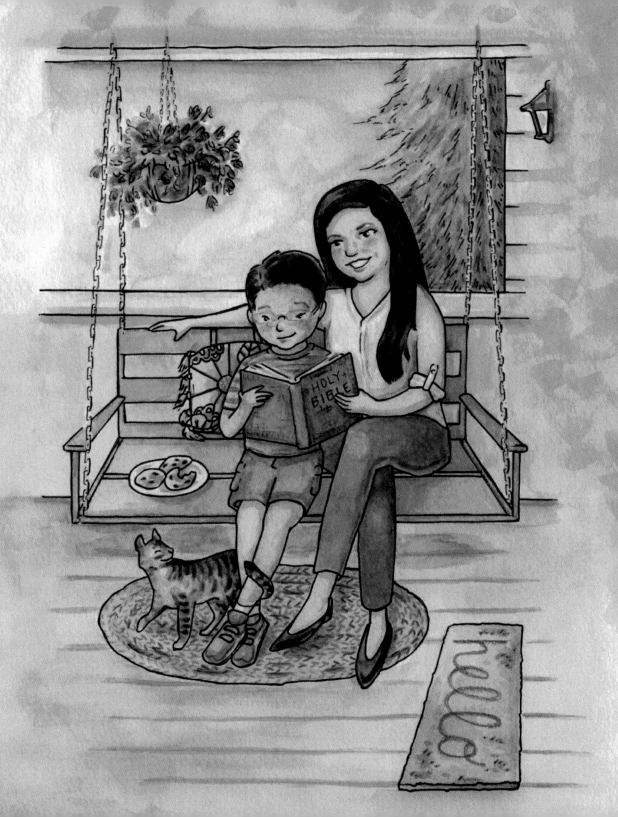

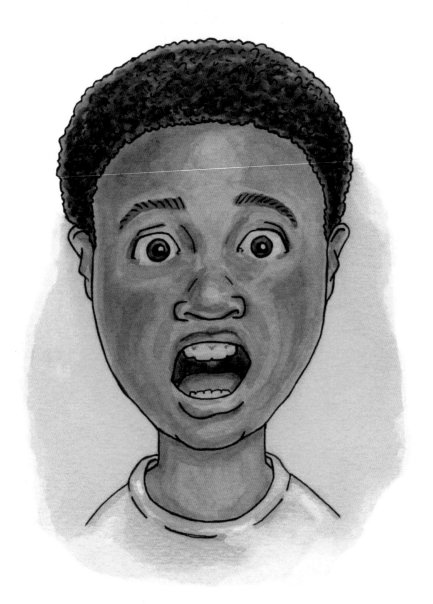

"WHAT!" Allen was so surprised! "Sometimes kids tease me because I am in a wheelchair. That hurts my feelings. I don't feel like praying for them!"

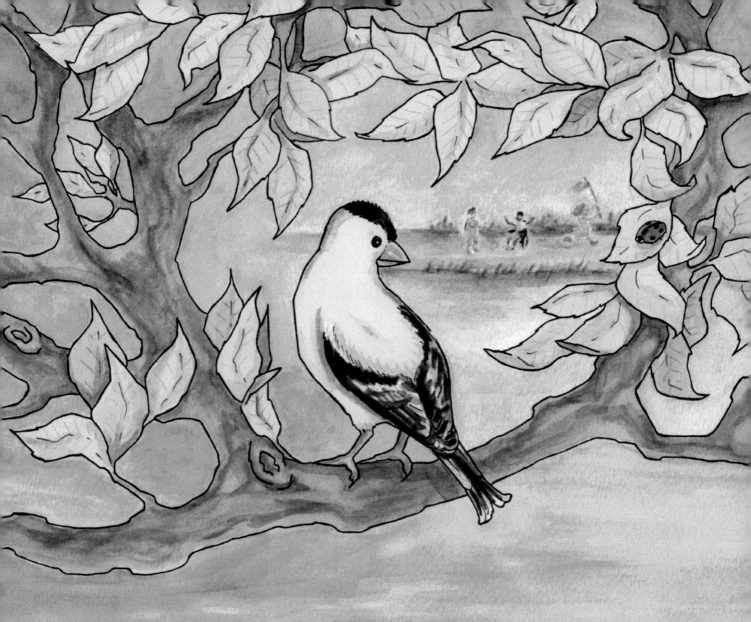

Harlow replied, "The more you pray for those
who are mean to you, the easier it is to forgive
them. If you obey God, He will bless you for it.
That's what Aunt Rebecca says."

Olive's face got as red as her hair as she shouted, "Ollie is in the river!"

Harlow assured her that Ollie was safe.

Ollie barked, saying hello to his friends while doing the doggie paddle. Beaver and Otter heard Ollie. They both swam as fast as they could to get to their friend. "Hi, Ollie," they both said at the same time.

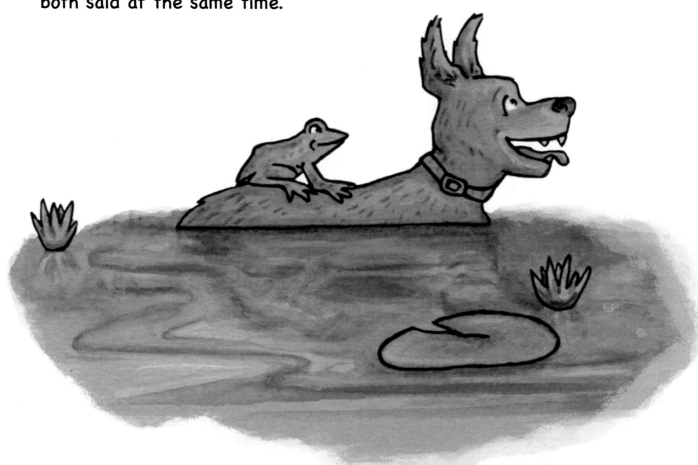

"Hey, Beaver. Can I ride on your tail?" Ollie asked.
"Yeah, jump on."

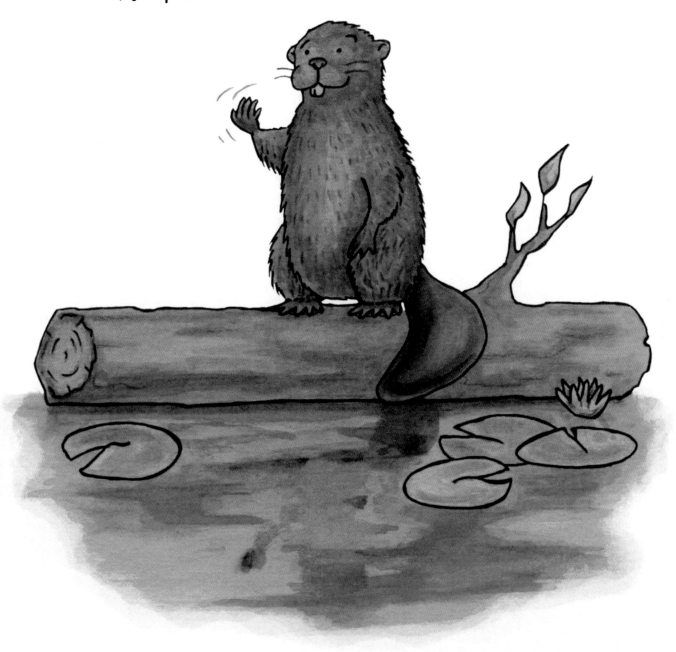

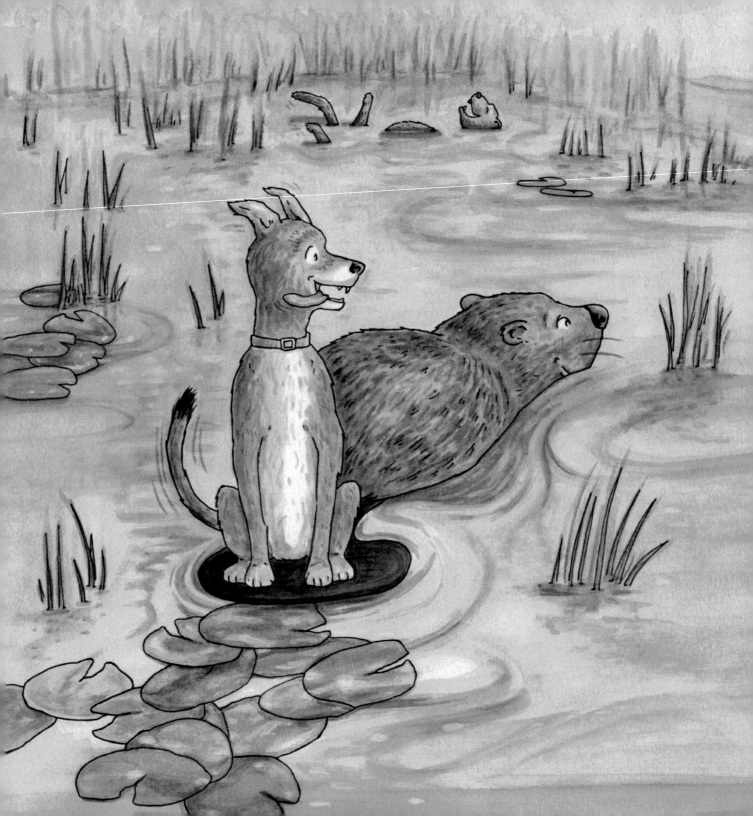

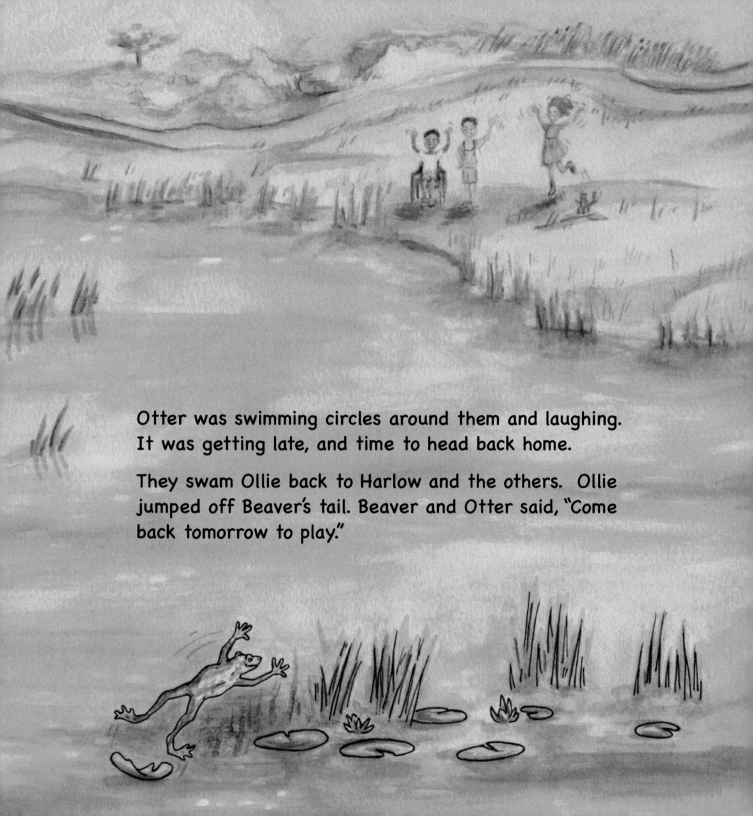

Otter was swimming circles around them and laughing. It was getting late, and time to head back home.

They swam Ollie back to Harlow and the others. Ollie jumped off Beaver's tail. Beaver and Otter said, "Come back tomorrow to play."

It seems like they are friends, too" Olive laughed.

Ollie, Beaver, and Otter looked at each other and smiled, "We are!"

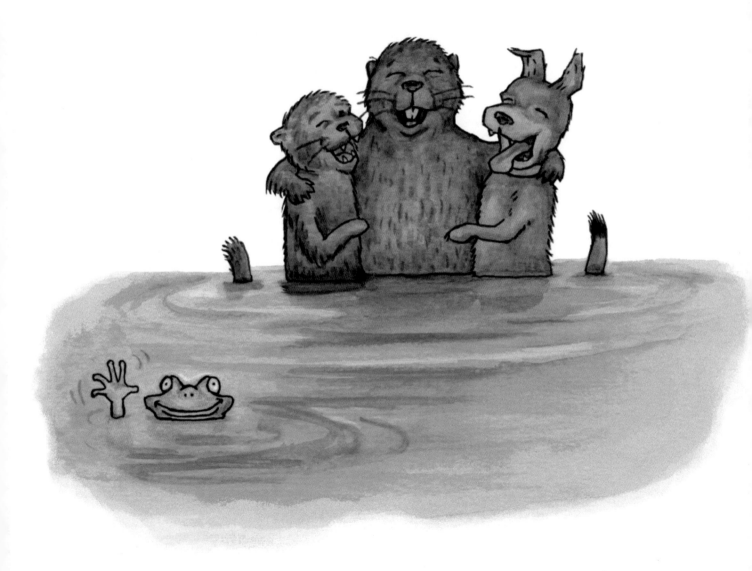

Beaver swooshed his tail and splashed everyone to say goodbye.

Everyone started laughing.

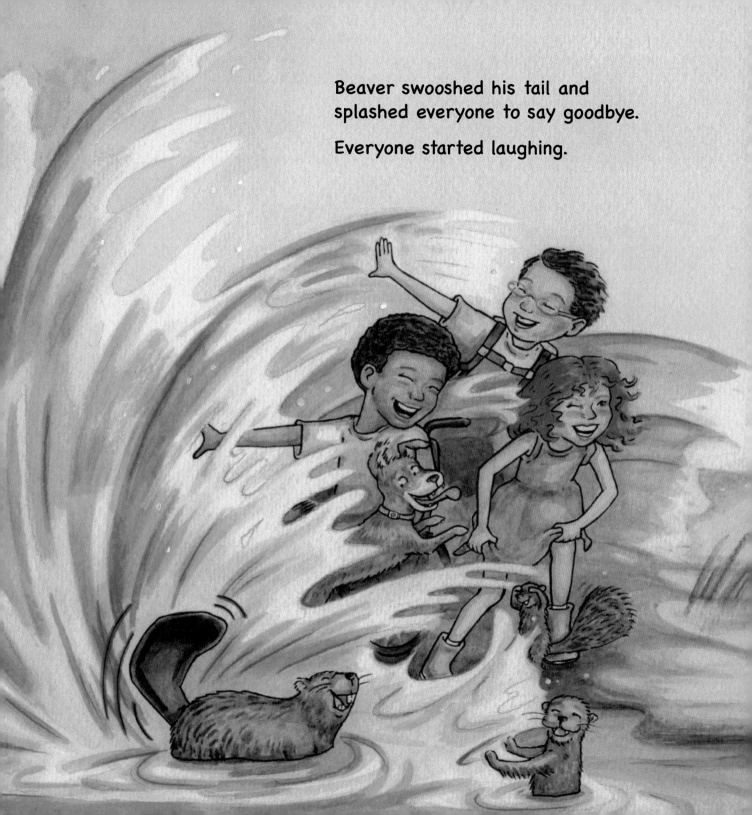

Do you know of someone
different from you?

If so, how can you make
them feel like they
belong?

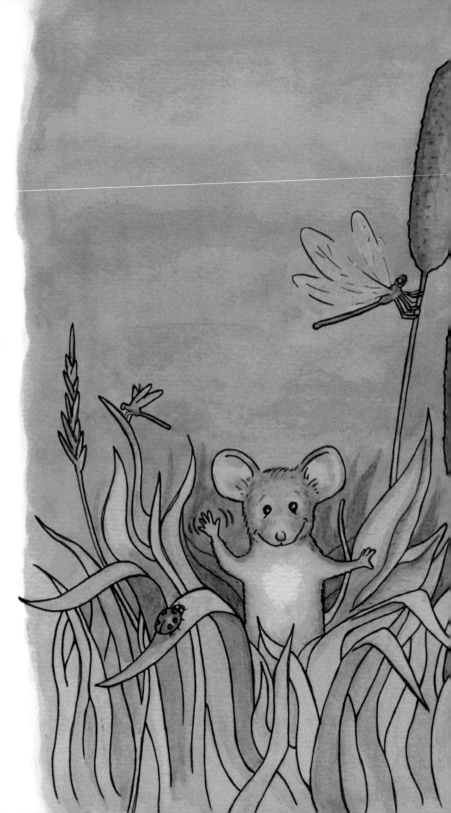

God did not make anyone the same.

We are all different, and WE ALL BELONG.

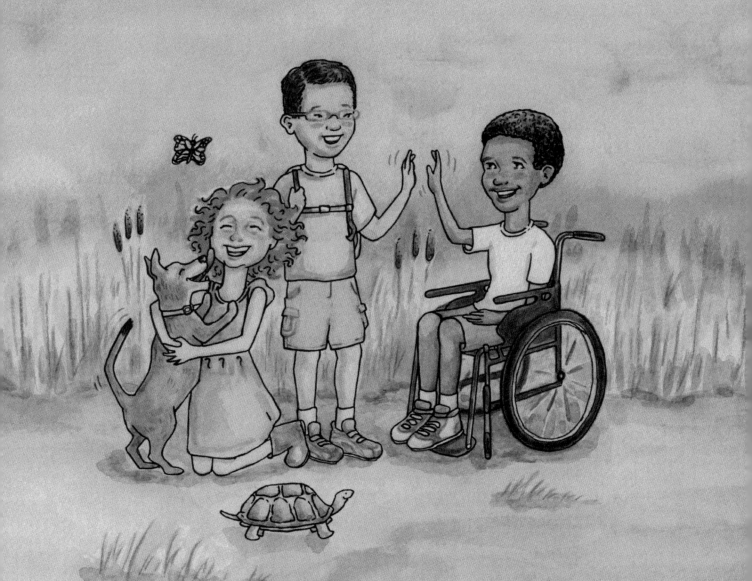

About the Author

Deborah K. Okon grew up on a dairy farm in northern Michigan. She retired 26 years from the Michigan Army National Guard as a Master Sergeant. Debbie also retired from the US Postal Service, working for 33 years. She still enjoys her career as a licensed massage therapist of 26 years.

Debbie loves spending mornings with Jesus and coffee and more coffee. Then time with family and friends. Debbie and her husband, George, live in Michigan. Together they have five children and four grandchildren.

Debbie is wearing red glasses to honor the memory of a special 5-year-old girl named Audrey.

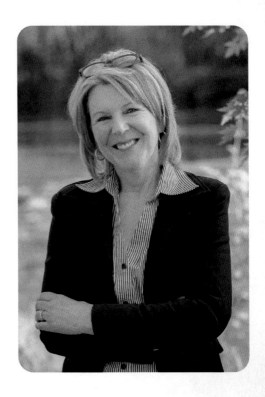

About the Illustrator

Halsey Mollhagen is a freelance illustrator and graduate of Kendall College of Art and Design.

Her artistic career includes a wide variety of creative projects. For over ten years, she has specialized in portraiture art. She is also the illustrator of **Never Play Checkers With a Leapfrog**, a poetry book written by Todd Day.

Halsey's illustrations bring endearing characters to the page in a playful and expressive style.

She resides in Grand Rapids, Michigan, with her husband and two young children.

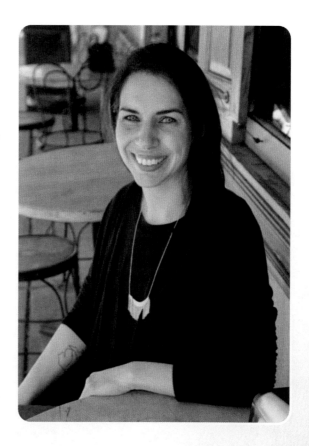

About Harlow

Harlow is a real person. If you would like to follow his adventures, please follow the links below:

Instagram: @whatshappening_harlow

Website: www.whatshappeningharlow.com

YouTube: youtube.com/whatshappeningharlow

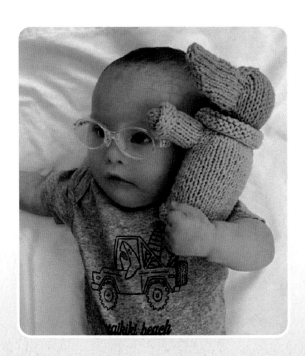

Acknowledgements

First and foremost, thanks to my primary source of strength and inspiration, my Lord and Savior, Jesus Christ.

My wonderful husband, George, you are invaluable. You are the most patient man I have ever known, next to my earthly father. Thank you for all your love and encouragement that carries me more than you realize.

Special thanks to my daughter, Rebecca, for your support and positive attitude. You saw that I was being "technically" challenged and stepped in to give me much-needed help. Very grateful for those extra trips to my house.

Many thanks to all who prayed for me!

Thank you, Pastor Dave Williams, Nicole Kelley-Korson, Cristel Phelps, Sandy, Jude, Miriam, and Leta O'Connor for helping me.

To Halsey Mollhagen for managing to capture my ideas on paper. Thank you for your willingness to assist and unite with me to complete this endeavor.

Special thanks to Harlow's cousins Halia, West, Simon, Nathan, and Otto. Simon, I heard you wore special socks to school to honor Harlow. That was so cool! Halia and West, Harlow loves playing with all the toys you give him.

Lastly, Donna Partow is a world-renowned author and speaker. I have been through military training. Now I have been through the "Jersey Girl's" coaching and mentorship Book Launch Training. They both challenged me to develop confidence, inner fortitude, and gratitude I will never forget. Many thanks!

Made in the USA
Las Vegas, NV
22 October 2024

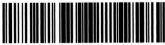